THE ULTIMA GUIDE TO PRILIGY(DAPOXETINE)

MW01233301

The Step by Step Guide for Treatment of Premature Ejaculation,Improve your Time and Control over Ejaculation to Last Longer in Bed and Maximize Sexual Pleasure

ISBN 978-1-0880-4278-6

Mattie Alphaman

TABLE OF CONTENT

CHAPTER 1

What exactly is the purpose of PRILIGY?

PRILIGY is a medication for premature ejaculation (PE) that is approved for use in male patients aged 18 to 64 years old who have all of the following conditions:

ejaculation in less than two minutes following vaginal penetration, most of the time with little stimulation and in advance of the man's desire to do so; and

considerable emotional anguish as well as difficulty in interpersonal relationships as a direct result of premature ejaculation (premature ejaculation causes problems for both the male and his partner); and insufficient control over ejaculation.

PRILIGY is a medication that is classified as a selective serotonin reuptake inhibitor (SSRI) and is also known as a urological treatment. Its active component is dapoxetine, and the drug is used to treat erectile dysfunction. PRILIGY shortens the amount of time it takes for you to ejaculate, which can help you gain more control over the process and feel less stressed about how quickly you ejaculate. It's possible that this will make you feel more satisfied with sexual encounters.

If you are unsure of why you have been given this medication, you should inquire about it with your primary care physician.

It's possible that your physician prescribed it for another purpose entirely.

This medication may only be obtained through a prescription from a medical professional.

CHAPTER 2
Before you take PRILIGY

When you must not take it

If you suffer from any of the following allergies, you should not use PRILIGY:

any pharmaceutical product that contains dapoxetine

any one of the components that are detailed at the bottom of this brochure.

The following are some examples of symptoms that may accompany an allergic reaction a feeling of difficulty breathing

coughing, chest tightness, or trouble breathing

a swelling of the cheeks, lips, tongue, or other regions of the body might be a sign of an allergic reaction.

hives, a rash, or itching on the surface of the skin.

Do not take PRILIGY:

If you are currently being treated for depression with a monoamine oxidase inhibitor (MAOI) medication or have taken an MAOI within the past 14 days, you should not use this medication (see Taking other medicines for examples of MAOIs). After you have stopped taking PRILIGY, you will have to wait a full week before beginning treatment with an MAOI.

if you are currently being treated with the antipsychotic medication thioridazine or if you have taken this medication in the past 14 days. After you have stopped using PRILIGY, you will have to wait a full week before beginning treatment with thioridazine.

if you are currently being treated for depression with a selective serotonin reuptake inhibitor (SSRI), as well as some other antidepressant medications and herbal remedies, or if you have been treated with any of these medications within the past 14 days. (for more examples of SSRIs and other medications used to treat depression, read our article on Taking other medications.) You will need to wait a full week before you can resume taking these drugs or herbal preparations after you have stopped taking PRILIGY.

if you are using certain medications for the treatment of fungal infections or drugs to treat HIV, you may experience side effects (see Taking other medicines for examples of these medicines).

In the event that you have a previous diagnosis of manic depression or severe depression

PRILIGY should not be taken by anybody who has a history of cardiac difficulties, including heart failure or issues with the heart's rhythm.

Do not use PRILIGY if you have moderate to severe liver issues.

If you have a history of dizziness, lightheadedness, or fainting due to a brief reduction in blood pressure, you should not use PRILIGY (Syncope).

PRILIGY should not be taken by anyone who is less than 18 years old or older than 65 years old.

It has not been determined whether or whether patients under the age of 18 or over the age of 65 would have any adverse effects.

If you are a female, you should not take PRILIGY.

Men who experience premature ejaculation have been the subject of research about the usage of PRILIGY. It has not been determined whether or not it is safe for use in females.

Lactose is present in this medication (a type of sugar). In the event that your physician has informed you that you have an intolerance to certain sugars, you should consult with your physician before using this medication.

Do not use this medication after the "best if used by" date that is marked on the package, or if the packaging is damaged in any way or shows symptoms of having been tampered with.

Return it to your pharmacist for disposal if it has beyond its expiration date or if it is damaged.

Talk to a medical professional if you are unsure about whether or not you should begin taking this medication.

Before you begin to take it, make sure you...

Before you begin taking this medication, your physician should conduct a test to ensure that your blood pressure does not drop too significantly when you rise up from a seated or laying down position after having been in either of those positions.

Tell your doctor if any of the following apply:

whether or whether you are allergic to any other medications, foods, preservatives, or colours.

It has not been determined that you are experiencing premature ejaculation.

You partake in the usage of recreational drugs like ecstasy and LSD. Combining these medications with PRILIGY might result in life-threatening side effects.

You may choose to use benzodiazepines like Valium or severe pain medications known as opioids. These other medications may amplify the sleepiness and lightheadedness caused by PRILIGY.

you consume alcohol. While using PRILIGY, you should avoid drinking alcohol since it might make you more susceptible to passing out.

You are currently receiving therapy for your depression.

You are now treating fungal infections using medicine in order to treat them.

Inform your physician if you now suffer from or have ever suffered from any of the following medical conditions:

a previous history of lightheadedness due to low blood pressure

difficulties with the heart and the blood vessels

bleeding tendencies

depression

passing out (see Things to be careful of)

do you ever consider killing yourself or
hurting yourself in any way?

mental health conditions, such as
schizophrenia

history of mania (high excitement,
hallucinations, trouble in focusing or being
quiet) or bipolar illness (severe mood
fluctuations) could develop one of these
conditions in the future.

epileptic convulsions (fits) or be
uncontrollable in their epilepsy

moderate or severe liver issues

serious renal issues

sexual problems, including erection
problems (sometimes called impotence). It
is unknown at this time whether or not
PRILIGY can make these situations more
worse.

difficulties with the eyes, such as glaucoma
(high pressure in the eye)

HIV

Before you start taking PRILIGY, you should discuss any of the following with your physician, especially if you haven't done so already.

CHAPTER 3

DRUG TO AVOID WHEN TAKING PRILIGY

Using many additional medications

Inform your primary care physician or your pharmacist if you are taking any additional medications, including over-the-counter medications that you may purchase from your local pharmacy, grocery store, or health food store.

There is a potential for PRILIGY and some medications to interact negatively with one another. These are the following:

Moclobemide, phenelzine, and tranylcypromine are examples of monoamine oxidase inhibitors (MAOIs), which are medications prescribed for the treatment of depression.

medications used to treat depression such as amitriptyline, citalopram, escitalopram, doxepin, fluoxetine, fluvoxamine, mianserin, mirtazapine, nortriptyline, paroxetine, sertraline, venlafaxine or vortioxetine.

triptans, as well as other drugs (for the treatment of migraines) (e.g. sumatriptan,)

the analgesic medication tramadol

lithium, a drug that is used to treat mood disorders

thioridazine is a medication that can be used to treat schizophrenia.

linezolid is an antibiotic that is utilized in the process of infection treatment.

Tryptophan is a supplement that can improve your mood and make it easier for you to fall asleep.

A natural remedy called St. John's wort, also known as hypericum perforatum

It is not recommended to use PRILIGY in conjunction with any of the medications or herbal preparations on the preceding list, nor should it be taken within 14 days after discontinuing these medications.

You will need to wait a full week before you may take any of these medications or herbal remedies after you have stopped taking PRILIGY.

PRILIGY and other medications have the potential to interact negatively with one another. These are the following:

medications that cause your blood to become less thick, such as warfarin

ketoconazole, itraconazole, and fluconazole are examples of antifungal drugs that are often used.

There are a few anti-HIV medications, such as ritonavir, saquinavir, and atazanavir, that are available.

medications that are used to treat high blood pressure and chest discomfort (angina), an enlarged prostate, or erectile dysfunction (impotence), as these medications have the potential to drop your blood pressure, maybe even when you stand up.

medications designed to reduce inflammation, such as ibuprofen and aspirin

Certain antibacterial medications, such as erythromycin and clarithromycin, are used to treat infections.

aprepitant, a medicine for treating
queasiness

grapefruit. Grapefruit juice should not be
consumed during the preceding 24 hours
after taking PRILIGY.

either narcotics (which are severe pain
medications) or benzodiazepines like
valium. These other medications may
amplify the sleepiness and lightheadedness
caused by PRILIGY.

alcohol. While using PRILIGY, you should
avoid drinking alcohol since it might make
you more susceptible to passing out.

If you are unsure whether or not you are taking any of these medications, you should see your physician or pharmacist.

There is a possibility that PRILIGY will interact with these medications, which might compromise its effectiveness. It's possible that you'll require a different dosage of your medications, or maybe an entirely new set of meds altogether.

It's possible that PRILIGY will interact with medications that aren't on this list, which might compromise how effectively it works. While you are taking this medication, your doctor and pharmacist have more information about other medications that you should avoid or use caution with.

CHAPTER 4

How to properly administer PRILIGY

Be sure to devote close attention to each and every one of your doctor's and the pharmacist's instructions.

There is a possibility that they will vary from the information that is presented in this booklet.

How much should I have?

A single tablet of 30 milligrams should be taken as needed, about one to three hours before engaging in sexual activity. This is the suggested dosage.

Take only one pill at a time, and never more than once per 24 hours.

How to deal with it

Take the pills as directed with at least one full glass of water. Swallow the tablets whole.

You can take PRILIGY with or without meals. Both are OK.

Grapefruit juice should be avoided for at least 24 hours before starting PRILIGY treatment.

Drinking grapefruit juice while taking this medication may result in a higher overall concentration of the drug in your body.

When should you take it?

When you feel the desire, take the pill around one to three hours before engaging in sexual activity.

When sexual activity is going to take place, you should only take PRILIGY when it's absolutely necessary. It is not designed to be used constantly on a daily basis.

Due to the increased risk of adverse effects as well as the absence of further benefit, you should not take more than one pill at a time every twenty-four hours.

In the event that you forget to take it.

It is not an issue if you forget to take PRILIGY because the medication should only be used when it is really necessary.

If you consume too much (overdose)

If you or someone else may have taken an excessive amount of PRILIGY, you should seek medical attention as soon as possible by contacting your primary care physician, the Poisons Information Centre at 13 11 26 (Australia), or going to the local hospital's Accident & Emergency department. Carry out these steps even if there are no indications that you are being harmed or poisoned.

It's possible that you require immediate medical assistance

A word of caution before you begin using PRILIGY: the medication may cause you to feel faint, dizzy, or lightheaded while you are taking it.

To assist in reducing the likelihood of this occurring:

When taking PRILIGY, be sure to drink at least one full glass of water with it.

If you are feeling dehydrated, you should not take PRILIGY (you do not have enough water in your body).

This could take place if:

You have gone between four and six hours without having anything to drink that contains water.

You have been perspiring for quite some time now.

You have a disease that manifests itself by giving you a fever, making you throw up, or making you feel unwell.

You have been drinking booze.

If you have symptoms such as feeling sick, feeling dizzy, light-headed, feeling weak, confused, sweaty, or an abnormal heart beat, or if you feel light-headed when you stand up, immediately lie down so that your head is lower than the rest of your body or sit down with your head between your knees until you feel better. If you have symptoms such as feeling sick, feeling dizzy, light-headed, feeling weak, confused, sweaty, or an abnormal heart beat, seek medical attention immediately. In the event that you pass out, this will prevent you from falling and injuring yourself.

After you have been seated or lying down for a significant amount of time, you should not immediately rise up.

If you feel dizzy or faint while taking this medication, you should avoid driving and using any equipment or machinery.

If you feel dizzy or faint while taking this medication, you should notify your doctor immediately.

Things that are required of you.

Make sure that your healthcare provider and pharmacist are aware that you are currently taking PRILIGY before beginning treatment with any new medication.

You should let any other medical professionals, including dentists and pharmacists, who treat you know that you are currently taking this medication.

Make sure to attend each and every one of your doctor's appointments so that your development may be monitored.

Have a conversation with your primary care provider before you stop taking this medication. It is possible that you will have trouble sleeping and feel disoriented if you stop taking it, even if you have not been taking it on a daily basis.

Things that you really must not do.

If your doctor has not instructed you to do so, do not use PRILIGY to treat any other symptoms or conditions.

Never share your medication with another person, even if they are suffering from the same ailment as you are.

Things that need to be watched out for

Take extreme caution if you plan on driving or operating machinery until you have a better idea of how PRILIGY will effect you.

Dizziness, lightheadedness, weariness, sleepiness, and even fainting have been reported by some patients after using this medication. Do not go behind the wheel of a vehicle, operate heavy machinery, or engage in any other activity that might put you or others in harm's way if you are experiencing any of these symptoms.

While you are under the influence of this medication, you should avoid drinking alcohol.

If PRILIGY is used at the same time as alcohol, the side effects of alcohol, such as sleepiness, dizziness, delayed reflexes, or impaired judgment, may be exacerbated.

Check to see whether you are dehydrated, which means that your body does not have enough water in it.

It is possible for this to happen if it has been four to six hours since the last time you drank anything, if you have been perspiring for an extended amount of time, or if you have an illness that involves fever, vomiting, or diarrhea.

It's possible that PRILIGY will make you faint. Your chances of passing out or getting hurt as a result of fainting can be reduced by the following:

At least one full glass of water should be consumed when taking PRILIGY.

If you start to feel faint, dizzy, lightheaded, sweaty, shaky, clammy, nauseous, or otherwise ill, lay down as soon as possible so that you don't injure yourself by falling when you're out of it and passing out.

After taking PRILIGY, ensure that you do not rise up too soon if you have been seated or lying down.

If you have any of these symptoms or any that are similar to them, you should avoid using machinery and driving.

CHAPTER 5
Side effects

If you are taking PRILIGY and do not feel well while you are taking it, you should inform your physician or pharmacist as soon as possible.

Although the majority of patients benefit from taking this medication, a small percentage of patients may experience undesirable side effects. Side effects are possible with every medication. They can be serious at times, but for the most part, they are just jokes. If you experience any of the potential adverse effects, you should seek immediate medical treatment.

Do not let the following lists of potential adverse effects frighten you. It's possible that none of these will happen to you.

Talk to your healthcare provider or pharmacist about any concerns or questions you might have.

Stop using PRILIGY and visit your doctor as soon as possible if any of the following apply to you:

You are incoherent (seizures)

if you have dizziness or fainting when you stand up, if you notice any changes in your mood, if you have any suicidal thoughts or ideas about hurting yourself, call 911 immediately.

Notify your primary care physician or your pharmacist if you observe any of the following and they cause you concern:

nausea

headache

dizziness

Notify your primary care physician as soon as you can if you observe any of the following symptoms:

symptoms such as passing out or feeling dizzy when standing (see While you are taking PRILIGY)

elevated levels of blood pressure

shaking, tingling, or a numbness in the extremities

vision that is not clear

eye strain and a buzzing sound in the ears

nasal congestion

diarrhea, stomach pain, dry mouth, vomiting, ingesting, intestinal gas, constipation, and bloating are all symptoms associated with gastrointestinal distress.

high levels of perspiration

drowsiness, lethargy, and excessive yawning

trouble paying attention and feeling what's going on. irritable

trouble falling or staying asleep

agitation, anxiousness, reduced sexual drive, melancholy, and apathy are all symptoms of depression.

abnormal dreams

Notify your primary care physician as soon as possible or go to the emergency department of the hospital closest to you if any of the following occur:

Symptoms indicate an allergic reaction, such as a rash, itching, or hives on the skin; wheezing, trouble breathing, or shortness of breath; swelling of the face, lips, tongue, or other regions of the body.

Notify your primary care physician or your pharmacist immediately if you discover anything that is making you feel ill.

There is a possibility that some people will have additional unlisted negative effects.

Following the use of PRILIGY Storage

Before it is time to take your medication, make sure that you keep the tablets in the original packaging.

If you remove the pills out of their packaging, they could not maintain their quality for as long.

You should store your pills in a place that is dry and cold, and the temperature should not exceed 25 degrees Celsius.

It is imperative that neither PRILIGY nor any other medication be kept in the bathroom or anywhere close to the sink. It is important that you do not leave it in the car or on a windowsill.

Some medications cannot be used if they have been exposed to heat or moisture.

Put it in a location where youngsters can't get to it.

Medications should be kept in a secure cabinet that is elevated at least one and a half meters from the ground and is covered with a lock.

Disposal

In the event that your physician instructs you to stop taking this medication or the expiration date has passed, consult your pharmacist to find out what you should do with any remaining medication.

Product description
What it looks like

The film-coated tablets of PRILIGY 30 mg are light gray in color, round, and are marked with the number "30" inside of a triangle on one side.

PRILIGY is available for purchase in blister packs that include either three or six pills.

Ingredients The active component of PRILIGY is dapoxetine hydrochloride, which comes in a dose of 30 milligrams.

Additionally, it has lactose monohydrate in it.

microcrystalline cellulose

croscarmellose sodium colloidal anhydrous silica

magnesium stearate

hypromellose

titanium dioxide iron oxide oxide of ferric black yellow \striacetin

This medication does not have any azo dyes, sugar, gluten, or tartrazine in its formulation.

THE END

CPSIA information can be obtained
at www.ICGtesting.com
Printed in the USA
LVHW081112250822
726654LV00013B/972